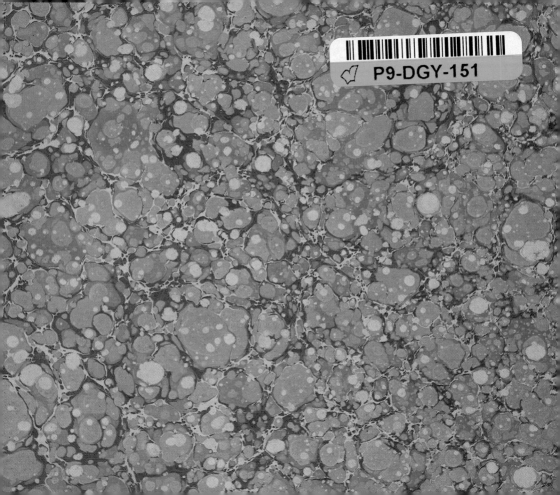

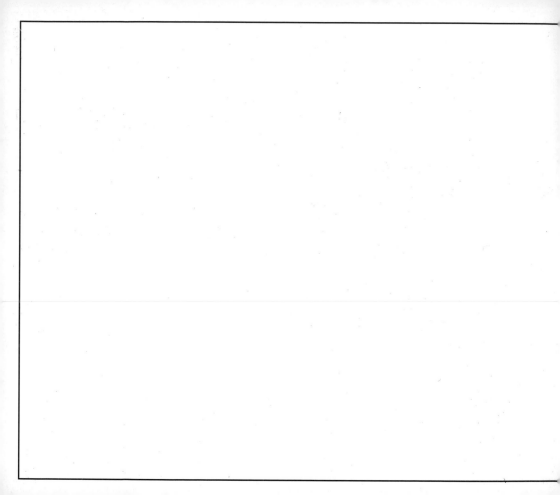

Cat's Companion
Anthology

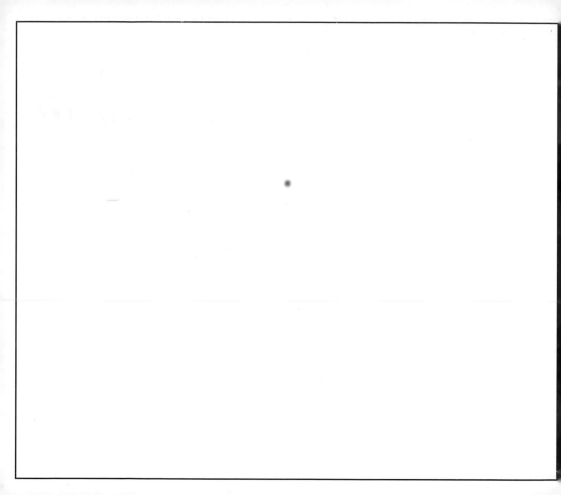

Cat's Companion
Anthology

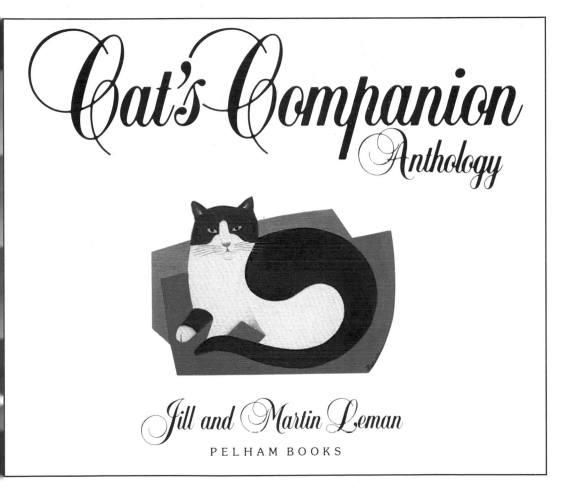

Jill and Martin Leman

PELHAM BOOKS

This book is a companion to

The Perfect Cat

also published by Pelham Books.

First published in Great Britain in 1986 by
Pelham Books Ltd, 27 Wrights Lane, London W8 5TZ
Reprinted 1987

ISBN 0 7207 1667 5

Printed and bound in Italy by New Interlitho

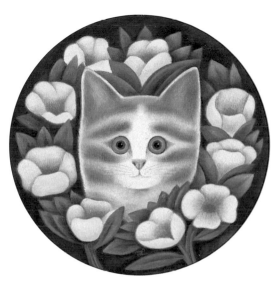

O lovely Pussy! O Pussy, my love,
What a beautiful Pussy you are,
     You are,
     You are!
What a beautiful Pussy you are!

Edward Lear

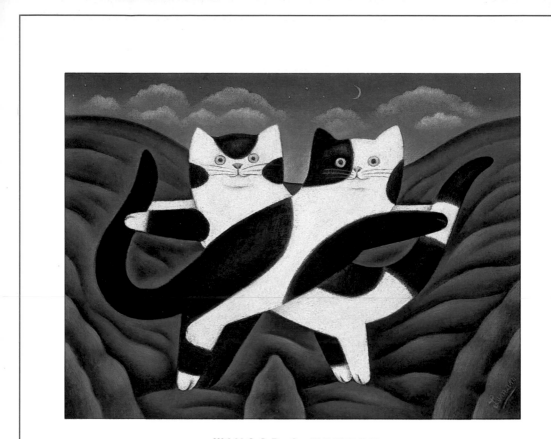

WINSOR & NEWTON

Jellicle Cats come out tonight,
Jellicle Cats come one come all:
The Jellicle Moon is shining bright –
Jellicles come to the Jellicle Ball.

Jellicle Cats are black and white,
Jellicle Cats are rather small;
Jellicle Cats are merry and bright,
And pleasant to hear when they caterwaul.
Jellicle Cats have cheerful faces,
Jellicle Cats have bright black eyes;
They like to practise their airs and graces
And wait for the Jellicle Moon to rise.

Jellicle Cats develop slowly,
Jellicle Cats are not too big;
Jellicle Cats are roly-poly,
They know how to dance a gavotte and a jig.
Until the Jellicle Moon appears
They make their toilette and take their repose:
Jellicles wash behind their ears,
Jellicles dry between their toes.

Jellicle Cats are white and black,
Jellicle Cats are of moderate size;
Jellicles jump like a jumping-jack,
Jellicle Cats have moonlit eyes.
They're quiet enough in the morning hours,
They're quiet enough in the afternoon,
Reserving their terpsichorean powers
To dance by the light of the Jellicle Moon.

Jellicle Cats are black and white,
Jellicle Cats (as I said) are small;
If it happens to be a stormy night
They will practise a caper or two in the hall.
If it happens the sun is shining bright
You would say they had nothing to do at all:
They are resting and saving themselves to be right
For the Jellicle Moon and the Jellicle Ball.

T. S. Eliot · The Song of the Jellicles

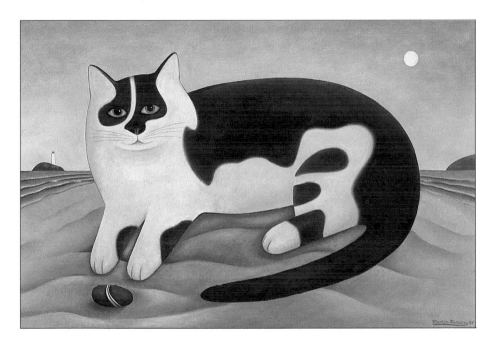

MERLIN

To assume a cat's asleep
is a grave mistake.
He can close his eyes and keep
both his ears awake.

Aileen Fisher · Half Asleep

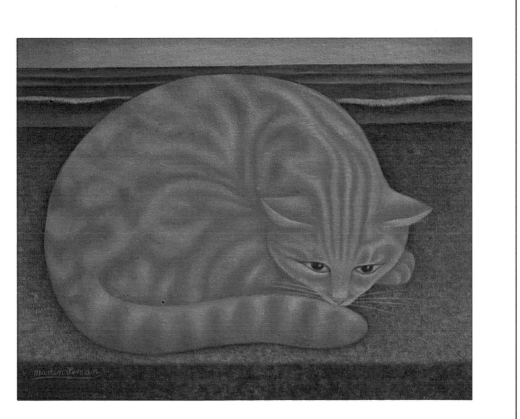

ROCKHOUSE FRED

I have a cat: I call him Pumpkin,
A great fat furry purry lumpkin.
Hi-dee-diddle hi-diddle dumpkin.

He sleeps within my bed at night,
His eyes are Mephistopheles-bright:
I dare not look upon their blight.

He stalks me like my angry God,
His gaze is like a fiery rod:
He dines exclusively on cod.

Avaunt, you creeping saviour-devil,
Away with thy angelic evil!

Stevie Smith · The Hound Puss

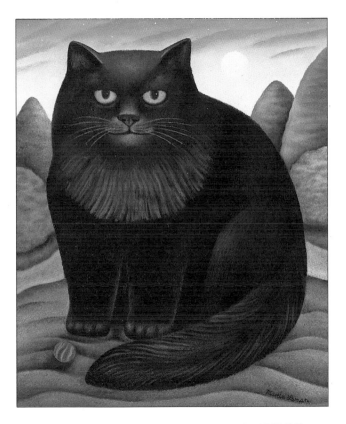

REVEREND WENCESLAS MUFF

Hear our prayer, Lord, for all animals,
May they be well-fed and well-treated and happy:
Protect them from hunger and fear and suffering:
And, we pray, protect specially, dear Lord,
The little Cat who is the companion of our home,
Keep her safe as she goes abroad,
And bring her back to comfort us.

Anon · An old Russian prayer

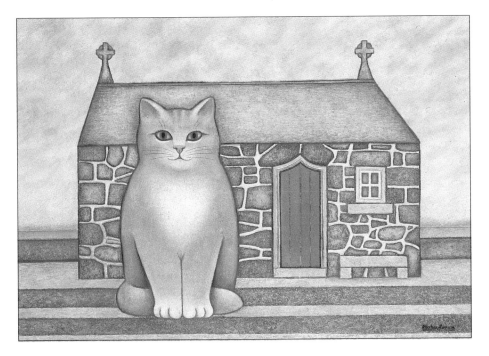

NICHOLAS

You're black and sleek and beautiful
What a pity your best friends won't tell you
Your breath smells of Kit-E-Kat.

Adrian Henri · Cat Poem

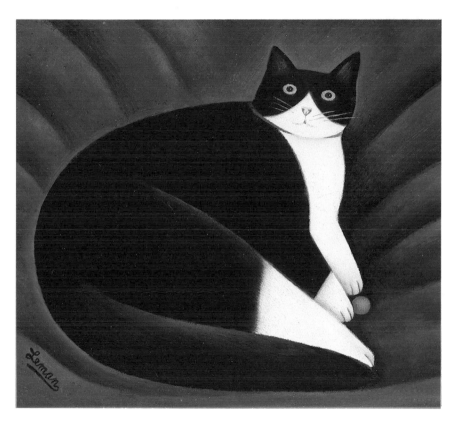

PERCY

Listen, Kitten,
Get this clear;
This is my chair,
I sit here.

Okay, Kitty,
We can share;
When I'm not home,
It's your chair.

Listen Tom Cat,
How about
If I use it
When you're out?

Richard Shaw · Squatter's Rights

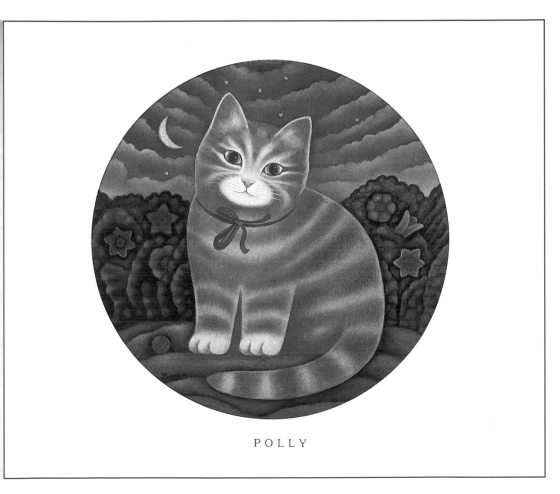

POLLY

I am not alone in the room:
   A bright intelligence
Watches the fire in the gloom
   Of Winter's imminence;

Wisdom it has from of yore
   Touching all things that concern it,
And all that I know of its lore
   Is that I shall never learn it.

Lord Dunsany · The Cat

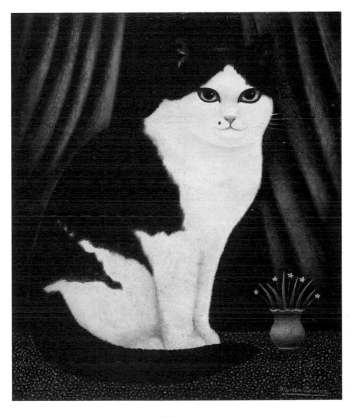

SPOT

Cats sleep fat and walk thin.
Cats, when they sleep, slump;
When they wake, pull in –
And where the plump's been
There's skin.
Cats walk thin.

Cats wait in a jump,
Jump in a streak.
Cats, when they jump, are sleek
As a grape slipping its skin –
They have technique.
Oh, cats don't creak.
They sneak.

Cats sleep fat.
They spread comfort beneath them
Like a good mat,
As if they picked the place
And then sat.
You walk around one
As if he were the City Hall
After that.

Rosalie Moore · Catalogue

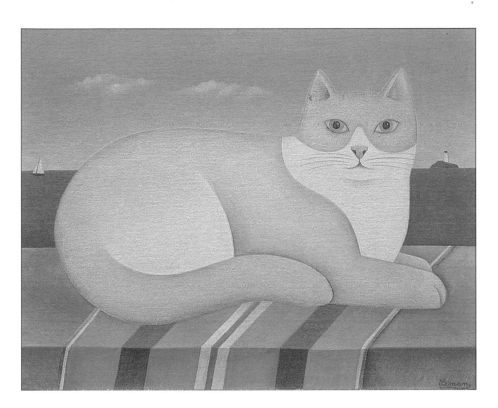

AMBROSE

Cat sentimentality is a human thing. Cats
are indifferent, their minds can't comprehend
the concept 'I shall die', they just go on living.
Death is more foreign to their thought than
to us the idea of a lime-green lobster. That's
why holding these warm containers of purring fur
is poignant, that they just don't know.
Life is in them, like the brandy in the bottle.

One morning a cat wakes up, and doesn't feel
disposed to eat or wash or walk. It doesn't panic
or scream: 'My last hour has come!' It
simply fades. Cats never go grey at the edges
like us, they don't even look old. Peter Pans,
insouciant. No wonder people identify with cats.

Gavin Ewart · Sonnet: Cat Logic

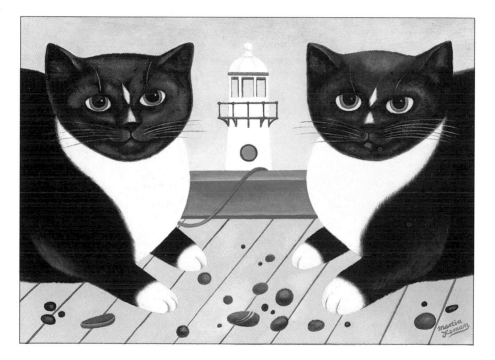

HUNTLEY & PALMER

It's very hard to be polite
     If you're a cat.
When other folks are up at table
Eating all that they are able,
You are down upon the mat
     If you're a cat.

You're expected just to sit
     If you're a cat.
Not to let them know you're there
By scratching on the chair,
Or a light, respected pat
     If you're a cat.

You are not to make a fuss
     If you're a cat.
Tho' there's fish upon the plate
You're expected just to wait,
Wait politely on the mat
     If you're a cat.

Anon · Under-the-table manners ·

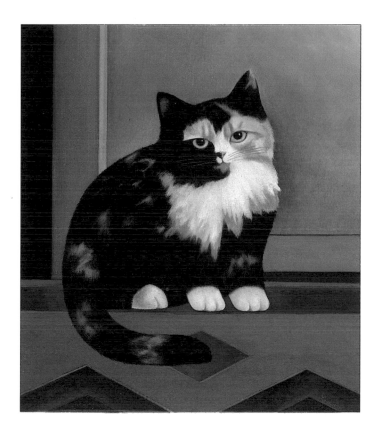

SCRUFFTY

Johnny is a long-haired Blue,
Looks a gentleman to you.
But his Ma was black and white,
Loved a dustbin, loved a fight;
And her little orphan boy,
Dressed up à la Fauntleroy,
Brushed and combed to look the part,
Has a wicked alley heart;
Swipes a titbit, smites a foe
With a fierce and expert blow;
Hands a deadly sock to those
Who interfere with his repose;
Circles round, intent to slog,
Any inoffensive dog;
Is profuse in phrases terse
And turns a ready, witty curse.
Yet he's a taking little brute,
The Bruiser in his ritzy suit.

Ruth Pitter · Three cheers for the black, white and blue.

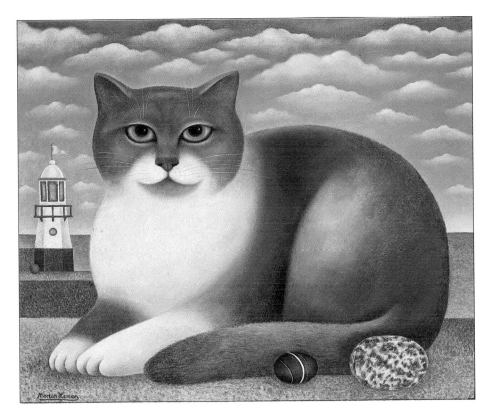

DELABOLE

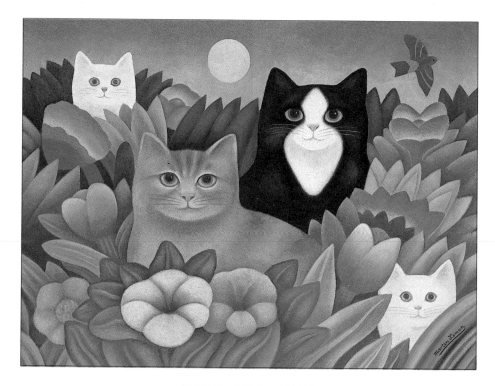

HIDE AND SEEK

A small wind
blows across the hedge
into the yard.
The cat cocks her ears
– multitudinous rustling
and crackling all round –
her pupils dwindle
to specks in
her yellow eyes
that stare first upward
and then on every side
unable to single out
any one thing

to pounce on,
for all together
as if orchestrated,
twigs, leaves,
small pebbles, pause
in their shifting,
their rubbing
against each other.

She is still listening
when the wind is already
three gardens off.

Thom Gunn · The cat and the wind

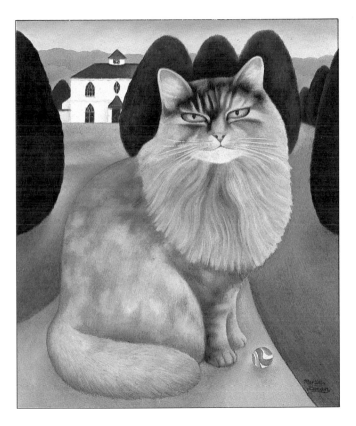

GLORIA

Always well-behaved am I,
Never scratch and never cry;
Only touch the diner's hand,
So that he can understand
That I want a modest share
Of the good things that are there.
If he pay but scanty heed
To my little stomach's need,
I beg him with a mew polite
To give me just a single bite.
Greedy though that diner be,
He will share his meal with me.

Antoinette Deshoulieres · Politeness Counts

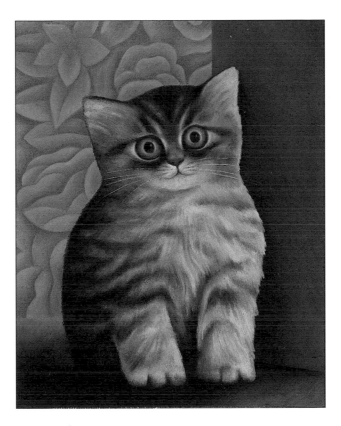

SWEET PEA

Come, my fine cat, against my loving heart;
Sheathe your sharp claws, and settle.
And let my eyes into your pupils dart
Where agate sparks with metal.

Now while my fingertips caress at leisure
Your head and wiry curves,
And that my hand's elated with the pleasure
Of your electric nerves,

I think about my woman – how her glances
Like yours, dear beast, deep-down
And cold, can cut and wound one as with lances;

Then, too, she has that vagrant
And subtle air of danger that makes fragrant
Her body, lithe and brown.

Pierre Charles Baudelaire · The Cat

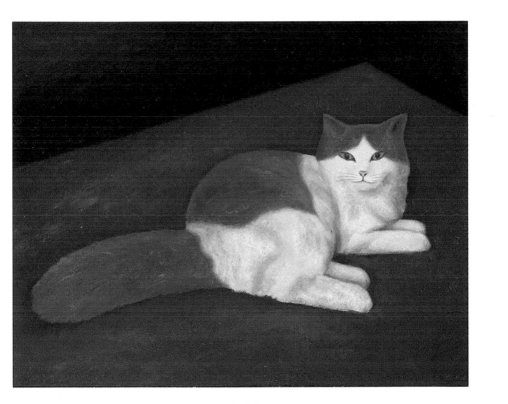

TOPAZ

In a dark garden, by a dreadful tree,
The Druid Toms were met. They numbered three,
Tab Tiger, Demon Black, and Ginger Hate.
Their forms were tense, their eyes were full of fate;
Save the involuntary caudal thrill,
The horror was that they should sit so still.
An hour of ritual silence passed: then low
And marrow-freezing, Ginger moaned 'OROW',
Two horrid syllables of hellish lore,
Followed by deeper silence than before.
Another hour, the tabby's turn is come;
Rigid, he rapidly howls 'MUM MUM MUM';
Then reassumes his silence like a pall,
Clothed in negation, a dumb oracle.
At the third hour, the black gasps out 'AH BLURK!'
Like a lost soul that founders in the murk;
And the grim, ghastly, damned and direful crew
Resumes its voiceless vigilance anew.
The fourth hour passes. Suddenly all three
Chant 'WEGGY WEGGY WEGGY' mournfully,
Then stiffly rise, and melt into the shade,
Their Sabbath over, and their demons laid.

Ruth Pitter · Quorum Porum*   *Porum: Genitive plural of 'Puss'

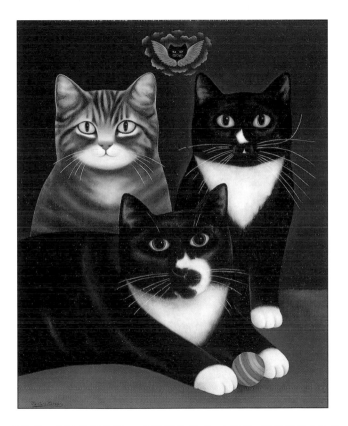

ZOË, MICKEY, SMUDGE AND PUDDING

He has conceived of a Republic of Mice
and a door through the fire,
parables of the reinstatement
of his balls. But not this night.
Isn't there a storm in the light bulb,
condors circling the kittens' meals
on the television screen?
He heard once that people wearied of
each other to escape unhappiness.
In his lovely sufficiency
he will string up endless garlands
for the moon's deaf guardians.
Moving one paw out and yawning,
he closes his eyes. Everywhere
people are in despair. And he is dancing.

Peter Porter · My old cat dances

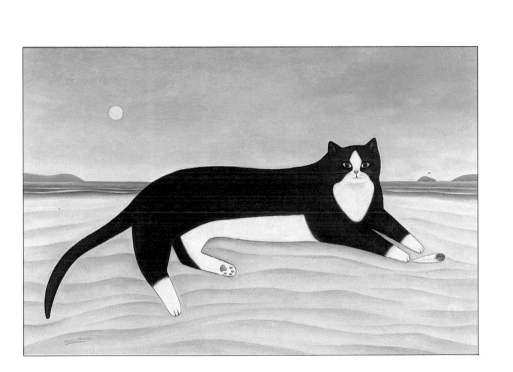

WALDO

Look at the gentle savage, monstrous gentleman
With jungles in his heart, yet metropolitan
As we shall never be; who – while his human hosts,
Afraid of their own past and its primaeval ghosts,
Pile up great walls for comfort – walks coquettishly
Through their elaborate cares, sure of himself and free
To be like them, domesticated, or aloof!
A dandy in the room, a demon on the roof,
He's delicately tough, endearingly reserved,
Adaptable, fastidious, rope-and-fibre nerved.
Now an accomplished Yogi good at sitting still
He ponders ancient mysteries on the window-sill,
Now stretches, bares his claws and saunters off to find
The thrills of love and hunting, cunningly combined.
Acrobat, diplomat, and simple tabby-cat,
He conjures tangled forests in a furnished flat.

Michael Hamburger · London Tom-cat

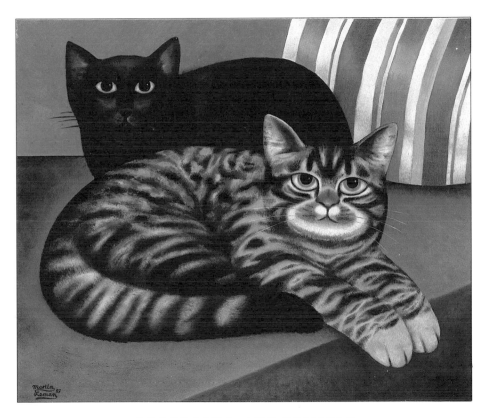

GOBBELINO AND SKIMBLE

When I remember Cornwall on
That last late summer trip,
I think of sun and blowing trees
And Cornish cream and coves and quays –
And Thomas of 'The Ship'!

He was a stray, the landlord said,
We think he's chosen well;
He likes the friendship and good fare
That visitors and 'locals' share
In this sea-shore hotel.

Dear Thomas! May you grow and thrive,
A 'Ship's Cat' through and through,
As back home, many a mile away,
The visitor who called one day
Is still remembering you!

Joan Pomfret · Cat Thomas

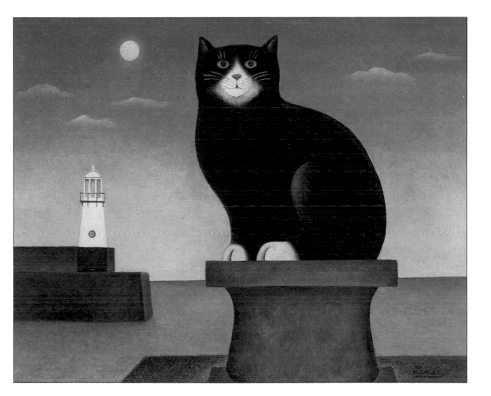

CAPTAIN

Our Cat
is the greatest thing on four legs
since Fred Astaire and Ginger Rogers.

Gavin Ewart · Broken-rhythm Haiku

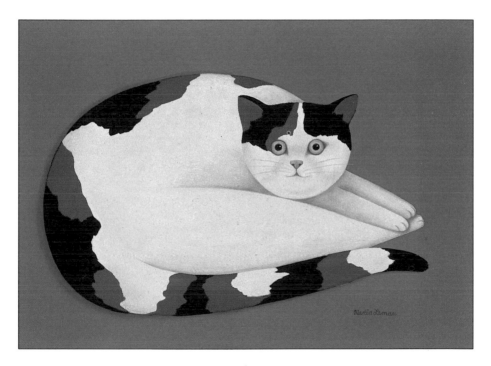

PATCH

When Tabby crouches by the fire,
  Primly agaze, her eyes are rings
Of agate flame: and strange desire
  Burns there, and old unholy things.

Surges on dream the lost Delight:
  And off she goes, careering down
The windy archways of the night,
  Afar on flying broomsticks blown.

R. W. D. Fuller · The Familiar

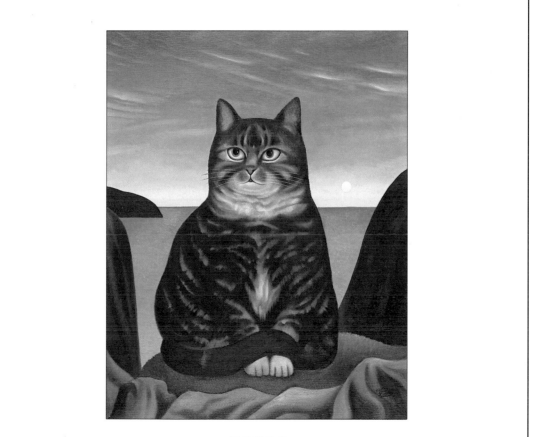

MOSES

He was a mighty hunter in his youth
At Polmear all day on the mound, on the pounce
For anything moving, rabbit or bird or mouse –
My cat and I grow old together.

After a day's hunting he'd come into the house
Delicate ears all stuck with fleas.
At Trenarren I've heard him sigh with pleasure
After a summer's day in the long-grown leas –
My cat and I grow old together.

When I was a child I played all day,
With only a little cat for companion,
At solitary games of my own invention
Under the table or up the green bay –
My cat and I grow old together.

Careful of his licked and polished appearance,
Ears like shell-whorls pink and transparent,
White plume waving proudly over the paths,
Against a background of sea and blue hydrangeas –
My cat and I grow old together.

A. L. Rowse · The White Cat of Trenarren

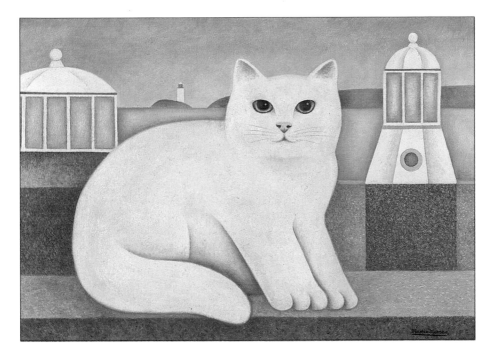

PEARL

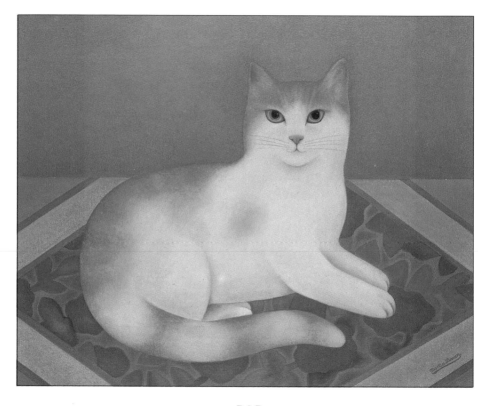

PIP

If I could
design an intimate
friend he would not
be covered in fur.

We would never
meet on the stairs
for a furry flirt
through the banister;
it is as nothing
to the real thing.

Our sharing
of the hearth
would be on
a different footing,
four feet –
two each side.

Sometimes, we could
eat in a restaurant
and I would purr
as I read the menu
with my green eyes
round in anticipation.
This would be more
exciting than discussing
a little bit of liver
in the kitchen.

An assignation in bed
would not begin
with the tip of a tail
walking round the edge,
like a sail appearing
on the edge of a field
by a river,
followed only by
a passionate affair
with one of my ankles
and a deep sleep.

Pamela Lewis · Feminine and Neuter

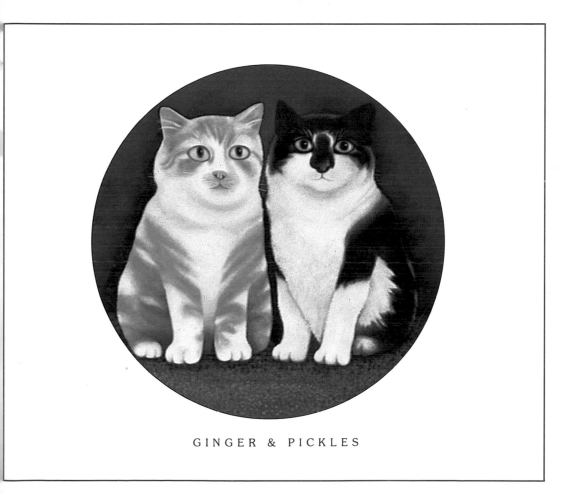

GINGER & PICKLES

Martin Leman would like to thank the many people who either commissioned or allowed him to paint their cats, especially the following:

Ann and John Curwin, GOBBELINO and SKIMBLE
Henrietta Winthrop and Paul Garside, SWEET PEA
Joan and Gil Gilbert, ROCK HOUSE FRED
Ina and Kevin Harris, ZOË, MICKEY, SMUDGE and PUDDING
Wendy and Robin Jacobs, SPOT
Peter Leigh, GLORIA
Sir Roy Strong, THE REVEREND WENCESLAS MUFF

For permission to use poems we should like to thank: Faber & Faber and Harcourt, Brace Jovanovich for 'The Song of the Jellicles' by T. S. Eliot from *Old Possum's Book of Practical Cats*. Robert Byrne, Teresa Skelton and Harper & Row, for 'Half-asleep' by Aileen Fisher from *Quotable Cats*. James MacGibbon, the Executor of the estate of Stevie Smith for 'The Hound Puss'. Adrian Henri for 'Cat Poem' from *The Mersey Sound Revised Edition*. Frederick Warne Inc. for 'Squatter's Rights' by Richard Shaw from *The Cat Book*. Rosalie Mander for 'The Cat' by Lord Dunsany and 'The Familiar' by R. W. D. Fuller from *CATegories* published by Weidenfeld & Nicolson. Gavin Ewart for 'Sonnet: Cat Logic' from *The Collected Ewart* published by Century Hutchinson and 'Broken-Rhythm Haiku' from *More Little Ones* published by Anvil Press. Century Hutchinson for 'Three Cheers for the black, white and blue', and 'Quorum Porum' from *Ruth Pitter on Cats*. Faber & Faber and Farrar, Straus & Giroux for 'The Cat and the wind' by Thom Gunn from *Passages of Joy*. Oxford University Press for 'My old cat dances' by Peter Porter from *Collected Poems*. Michael Hamburger for 'London Tom Cat' from *Collected Poems* published by Carcanet Press. Blackwood, Pillans & Wilson for 'The White Cat of Trenarren' from *A Life* by A. L. Rowse. Every effort has been made to trace the copyright owners of the material used in this anthology. The editor and publishers apologise for any omissions and would be pleased to hear from those whom they were unable to trace.

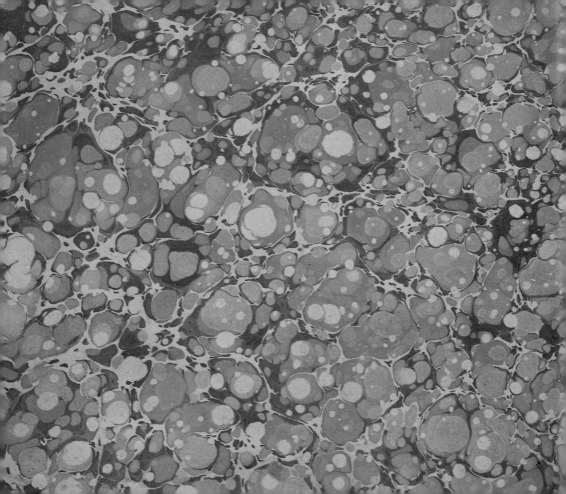